# KIDNEY DISEASE DIET FOR SENIORS ON STAGE 3

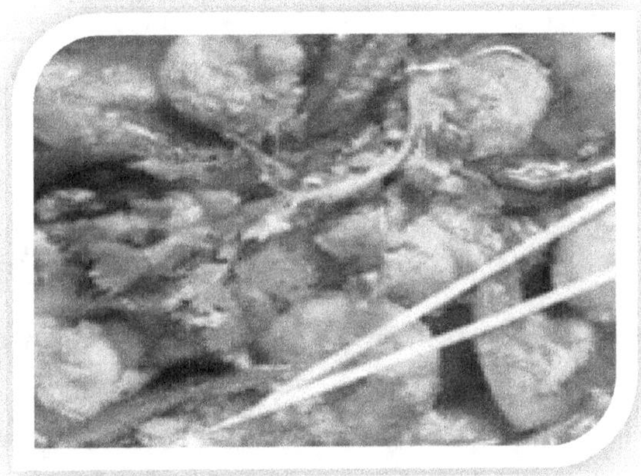

Delicious and Nutritious Recipes with Low-Sodium, Low-Potassium, and Low-Phosphorus, Along with a 30-Day Meal Plan for Seniors on a Restricted Diet

Dr. Linda B. Allen

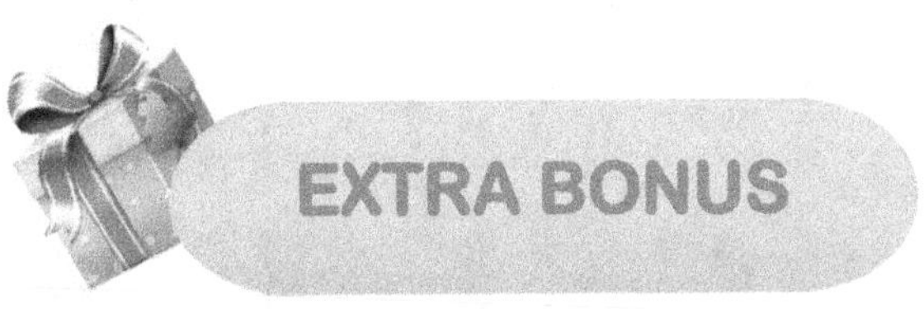


## BONUS NO. 1

### WEEKLY MEAL JOURNAL/PLANNER

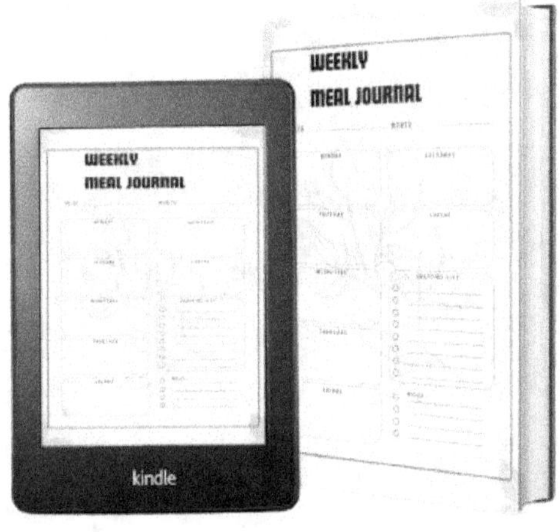


## BONUS NO.2

### TIPS FOR SUSTAINING A HEALTHY DIET WITH KIDNEY DISEASE

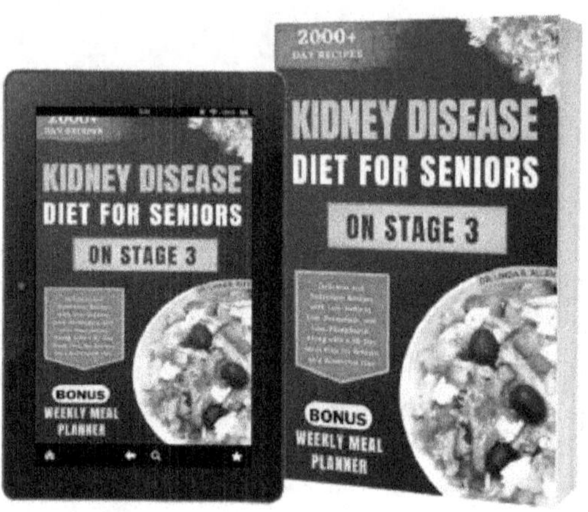

2000+
DAY RECIPES
KIDNEY DISEASE
DIET FOR SENIORS
ON STAGE 3
BONUS
WEEKLY MEAL
PLANNER
KIDNEY DISEASE
DIET FOR SENIORS
ON STAGE 3
BONUS
WEEKLY MEAL
PLANNER

# TABLE OF CONTENTS

# INTRODUCTION

In the realm of health and wellness, few elements wield as much influence as the food we consume. As a Doctor specializing in nutrition and dietetics, my journey has been one of steadfast commitment to unraveling the intricate relationship between what we eat and how it affects our well-being. Today, I am honored to present a labor of love and expertise: the "Kidney Disease Diet for Seniors on Stage 3."

This book encapsulates not just a compilation of recipes and meal plans but a profound understanding born from years of clinical experience and a deeply personal journey. My venture into the world of nutritional guidance emerged not solely from academic pursuits but from a poignant chapter in my life – the story of my cherished senior sister confronting stage 3 kidney disease.

Witnessing her battle became the impetus for delving deeper into the intricate nuances of kidney health. It was a journey marked by tireless research, endless consultations, and, above all, the pursuit of crafting a resource that would resonate with those facing similar challenges.

This book is an amalgamation of knowledge gleaned from helping countless individuals navigate the complexities of kidney disease. Its foundation rests on the principles of informed dietary choices tailored specifically for seniors managing stage 3 kidney disease. Within these pages lie the culmination of not just my professional insights but also the collective experiences of individuals whose lives I've had the privilege to touch.

At its core, this book is a beacon of hope for seniors grappling with kidney disease, a testament to the transformative power of food as medicine. It is a guide meticulously curated to navigate the dietary intricacies imposed by stage 3 kidney disease, offering not only sustenance but also flavor, variety, and a renewed sense of culinary delight.

## What Does This Book Offer?

This comprehensive guide is meticulously structured to address the multifaceted challenges that accompany kidney disease in seniors. It encompasses:

**1. Understanding Kidney Disease:** Delve into the nuances of stage 3 kidney disease – its symptoms, causes, and the critical role that diet plays in managing this condition. Gain insights into the significance of specific dietary restrictions such as low-sodium, low-potassium, and low-phosphorus foods.

**2. Tailored Nutritional Guidance:** Unlock the secrets of crafting a diet that promotes kidney health. Learn practical strategies and meal planning techniques designed to optimize nutrition while adhering to the dietary restrictions essential for managing stage 3 kidney disease.

**3. Delicious and Nutritious Recipes**: Explore a treasure trove of recipes thoughtfully curated to align with the dietary needs of seniors with kidney disease. From tantalizing breakfast options to satisfying lunch and dinner ideas, discover flavorful yet kidney-friendly meals that prioritize both taste and nutrition.

**4. 30-Day Meal Plan:** Embark on a guided culinary journey with a meticulously designed 30-day meal plan. This plan takes the guesswork out of meal preparation, offering a structured roadmap to support seniors in adhering to their dietary requirements without compromising on flavor or variety.

This book is not merely a compendium of recipes; it is a testament to empowerment through knowledge. It seeks to arm seniors and their caregivers with the tools necessary to navigate the dietary maze posed by kidney disease, fostering a sense of autonomy and well-being.

In the course of my practice, I have been privileged to witness remarkable transformations – individuals regaining control of their health and vitality through mindful dietary modifications. The stories of resilience, the joy of newfound culinary experiences, and the tangible improvements in health outcomes continue to fuel my dedication to empowering individuals on their path to wellness.

In essence, this book is a culmination of these experiences, a heartfelt endeavor to provide solace, guidance, and a renewed sense of culinary adventure to seniors navigating the complexities of stage 3 kidney disease.

Join me in this journey toward enhanced well-being, where the plate becomes a canvas for nurturing health and savoring life.

# Understanding Kidney Disease in Seniors:

Understanding kidney disease in seniors, particularly in its stage 3 manifestation, involves a nuanced comprehension of renal function, the progression of the disease, its impact on health, and the pivotal role that diet plays in managing this condition. Kidneys, those unassuming bean-shaped organs nestled in our lower back, serve as the body's filtration system, removing waste and excess fluids from the bloodstream, maintaining a balance of electrolytes, and regulating blood pressure.

## Overview of Stage 3 Kidney Disease:

Stage 3 kidney disease signifies a moderate decline in kidney function, typically categorized by a glomerular filtration rate (GFR) between 30-59 milliliters per minute. In this phase, the kidneys begin to exhibit reduced efficiency in filtering waste and excess fluids, leading to a buildup of toxins in the bloodstream. It's a critical juncture where proactive management becomes pivotal in slowing the progression of the disease and mitigating its associated complications.

# Understanding Kidney Disease in Seniors:

Seniors, due to the natural aging process, are more susceptible to kidney disease. Factors such as reduced kidney function over time, the cumulative impact of chronic conditions like hypertension or diabetes, and the use of certain medications contribute to an increased vulnerability. However, kidney disease often remains asymptomatic in its early stages, making regular screenings imperative for early detection and intervention.

The symptoms of kidney disease can be subtle initially, manifesting as fatigue, changes in urine output, swelling in extremities, or difficulty concentrating. As the disease progresses, symptoms may intensify, leading to complications like anemia, bone disease, fluid retention, and an increased risk of cardiovascular issues.

# Importance of Diet in Managing Kidney Health:

Diet assumes paramount importance in managing kidney health, especially in stage 3 kidney disease.

A meticulously crafted diet can alleviate the strain on compromised kidneys, slowing the progression of the disease and enhancing overall well-being.

**Managing Sodium Intake:** Sodium, found abundantly in processed and packaged foods, can exacerbate fluid retention and increase blood pressure, placing added stress on the kidneys. Seniors with stage 3 kidney disease benefit immensely from a low-sodium diet, reducing the risk of edema and hypertension.

**Low-Potassium Foods:** Potassium, an electrolyte vital for nerve and muscle function, can accumulate in the bloodstream due to compromised kidney function. In stage 3 kidney disease, maintaining a balance by consuming low-potassium foods helps prevent heart irregularities and muscle weakness.

**Understanding Low-Phosphorus Diet:** Kidneys struggling with reduced function struggle to regulate phosphorus levels, leading to bone weakening and cardiovascular issues. Seniors with stage 3 kidney disease often benefit from limiting phosphorus-rich foods, emphasizing a diet that favors low-phosphorus alternatives.

**Protein Moderation:** While protein is crucial for bodily functions, excess protein can burden compromised kidneys. Seniors in stage 3 kidney disease often require a balanced approach to protein intake, ensuring adequate amounts without overwhelming the kidneys.

Crafting a diet that aligns with these principles becomes a cornerstone in managing kidney health. It demands a delicate balance between ensuring adequate nutrition and adhering to dietary restrictions imposed by the disease. Consulting with healthcare professionals, particularly registered dietitians or nutritionists specializing in renal health, proves instrumental in tailoring diets that optimize nutrition while mitigating the progression of stage 3 kidney disease in seniors.

# WHAT IS STAGE 3 KIDNEY DISEASE?

Stage 3 kidney disease marks a critical stage in the progression of renal impairment. To truly comprehend its nuances, it's essential to delve into what stage 3 kidney disease entails, the array of symptoms and indicators it presents, and the complex web of factors that increase the risk and contribute to its development.

**What is Stage 3 Kidney Disease?**

Stage 3 kidney disease represents a moderate decline in kidney function, typically indicated by a glomerular filtration rate (GFR) ranging from 30 to 59 milliliters per minute. This phase signifies a critical juncture where the kidneys begin to demonstrate reduced efficiency in filtering waste and excess fluids from the bloodstream. While it is considered a moderate stage, its implications for overall health and the progression of kidney dysfunction are significant.

## Symptoms and Indicators:

In its earlier stages, kidney disease often remains asymptomatic, making routine screenings imperative for early detection. However, as the disease progresses, an array of symptoms may manifest:

**Changes in Urination:** Individuals may notice alterations in urine output, such as increased frequency or changes in color, particularly darker urine.

**Swelling:** Edema or swelling, especially in the extremities like legs, ankles, and face, can occur due to fluid retention.

**Fatigue:** Persistent fatigue and weakness, often unrelated to exertion, may signal kidney dysfunction.

**Difficulty Concentrating:** Brain fog or difficulty concentrating may arise due to waste buildup in the bloodstream affecting cognitive function.

**Anemia:** Decreased production of red blood cells can lead to anemia, resulting in fatigue and weakness.

These symptoms may intensify as kidney function continues to decline, highlighting the importance of regular health check-ups, especially for individuals at risk.

# Causes and Risk Factors:

Understanding the causes and risk factors contributing to stage 3 kidney disease sheds light on its multifaceted nature:

**Chronic Conditions:** Underlying chronic conditions such as hypertension or high blood pressure and diabetes are primary contributors to kidney disease. Prolonged uncontrolled blood sugar levels or high blood pressure can damage blood vessels in the kidneys, impairing their function over time.

**Aging:** The natural aging process results in a gradual decline in kidney function. Seniors are more susceptible to kidney disease due to these age-related changes.

**Family History:** A family history of kidney disease or genetic predispositions can elevate the risk of developing kidney problems.

**Medications and Toxins:** Certain medications, especially if used over prolonged periods, can contribute to kidney damage. Additionally, exposure to environmental toxins or heavy metals can impact renal health.

**Smoking and Obesity:** Unhealthy lifestyle choices, such as smoking and obesity, significantly increase the risk of kidney disease. Smoking damages blood vessels, including those in the kidneys, while obesity contributes to conditions like diabetes and hypertension, exacerbating kidney complications.

**Other Conditions:** Certain autoimmune diseases, infections, and kidney infections (such as chronic pyelonephritis) can also lead to kidney damage if left untreated.

Navigating the labyrinth of causes and risk factors associated with stage 3 kidney disease underscores the need for proactive health management. Lifestyle modifications, regular screenings, and early intervention become pivotal in mitigating the risk and progression of kidney disease.

In essence, stage 3 kidney disease represents a pivotal phase in the spectrum of renal health. Its identification through understanding its symptoms, grasping the array of causes and risk factors, and the importance of proactive health management underscore the significance of early detection and intervention in preserving kidney function and overall well-being.

Navigating the dietary landscape for individuals grappling with stage 3 kidney disease necessitates a nuanced understanding of foods to include and avoid. Managing sodium intake, monitoring potassium levels, and comprehending the nuances of a low-phosphorus diet are pivotal in preserving kidney health and mitigating the progression of the disease.

## Managing Sodium Intake for Kidney Health:

Sodium, a prevalent component in numerous processed and packaged foods, plays a significant role in fluid balance and blood pressure regulation. However, for individuals with compromised kidney function, excessive sodium intake can exacerbate fluid retention and elevate blood pressure, placing added strain on the kidneys.

Opting for a low-sodium diet becomes imperative in managing stage 3 kidney disease. This entails minimizing the consumption of high-sodium foods such as processed meats, canned soups, certain condiments, and processed snacks.

Instead, emphasis should be placed on whole, fresh foods that are naturally low in sodium. Incorporating fresh fruits, vegetables, lean proteins, and whole grains while steering clear of high-sodium additives and processed foods can significantly aid in maintaining optimal fluid balance and blood pressure.

## Low-Potassium Foods for Stage 3 Kidney Disease:

Potassium, an electrolyte essential for nerve and muscle function, assumes a delicate balance in the context of kidney disease. Impaired kidney function can lead to an accumulation of potassium in the bloodstream, potentially causing heart irregularities and muscle weakness.

Managing potassium intake becomes paramount. Identifying and incorporating low-potassium foods into the diet is crucial. While many fruits and vegetables are high in potassium, opting for varieties that are lower in this electrolyte can help maintain a healthy balance. Examples include apples, berries, cabbage, cauliflower, and green beans.

Ensuring proper portion sizes and avoiding high-potassium foods like bananas, oranges, tomatoes, and potatoes can aid in controlling potassium levels and alleviating strain on the kidneys.

## Understanding Low-Phosphorus Diet for Seniors:

Phosphorus, a mineral abundant in various foods, plays a vital role in bone health and cell function. However, in the context of compromised kidney function, the kidneys struggle to regulate phosphorus levels, leading to potential complications such as bone weakening and cardiovascular issues.

A low-phosphorus diet becomes imperative for seniors managing stage 3 kidney disease. Limiting the consumption of high-phosphorus foods such as dairy products, nuts, seeds, whole grains, and certain meats is crucial. Instead, incorporating foods that are lower in phosphorus, such as rice, pasta, bread made from refined flour, and fresh fruits and vegetables, becomes pivotal in managing phosphorus levels in the bloodstream.

Careful consideration of portion sizes and a focus on fresh, whole foods while minimizing intake of high-phosphorus additives commonly found in processed foods contribute to effective management of phosphorus levels in the diet.

In essence, the intricate dance between managing sodium intake, monitoring potassium levels, and understanding the intricacies of a low-phosphorus diet forms the crux of dietary management for individuals navigating stage 3 kidney disease. It requires a concerted effort to strike a balance between optimal nutrition and adherence to dietary restrictions imposed by kidney disease, empowering individuals to proactively manage their health and well-being.

# Low-Sodium and Kidney-Friendly Breakfasts

## 1. Quinoa Breakfast Bowl

**Ingredients:**

- 1/2 cup quinoa, rinsed
- 1 cup unsweetened almond milk
- 1/2 teaspoon cinnamon
- 1 tablespoon chopped almonds
- 1 tablespoon fresh berries (blueberries, raspberries)
- 1 teaspoon honey or maple syrup (optional)

**Preparation:**

1. In a saucepan, combine quinoa and almond milk. Bring to a boil, then reduce heat, cover, and simmer for 15-20 minutes until quinoa is cooked and liquid is absorbed.
2. Stir in cinnamon and transfer the cooked quinoa to a bowl.

3.  Top with chopped almonds, fresh berries, and a drizzle of honey or maple syrup if desired.

**Portion Size:** 1 serving

**Nutritional Information (approximate):**

Calories: 300 kcal, Protein: 10g, Carbohydrates: 45g, Fiber: 6g, Sodium: 50mg

## 2. Veggie Omelette

**Ingredients:**

- 2 eggs
- 1/4 cup chopped bell peppers
- 1/4 cup chopped spinach
- 2 tablespoons diced tomatoes
- 1 tablespoon chopped onion
- 1 teaspoon olive oil
- Salt-free seasoning blend
- Fresh herbs for garnish (optional)

**Preparation:**

1.  In a bowl, beat the eggs and set aside.
2.  Heat olive oil in a non-stick skillet over medium heat. Add onions and bell peppers, sauté until slightly softened.
3.  Add spinach and tomatoes, cook for another minute.
4.  Pour the beaten eggs over the veggies in the skillet. Cook until the omelette sets, then fold it in half.
5.  Season with salt-free seasoning blend and garnish with fresh herbs if desired.

**Portion Size:** 1 omelette

**Nutritional Information (approximate):**

Calories: 180 kcal, Protein: 12g, Carbohydrates: 6g, Fiber: 2g, Sodium: 70mg

## 3. Overnight Chia Pudding

**Ingredients:**

- 2 tablespoons chia seeds
- 3/4 cup unsweetened almond milk
- 1/4 teaspoon vanilla extract
- 1/2 cup sliced strawberries
- 1 tablespoon chopped walnuts

**Preparation:**

1. In a bowl, mix chia seeds, almond milk, and vanilla extract. Give it a good stir, then refrigerate for the entire night.
2. In the morning, top the chia pudding with sliced strawberries and chopped walnuts before serving.

**Portion Size:** 1 serving

**Nutritional Information (approximate):**

Calories: 220 kcal, Protein: 6g, Carbohydrates: 18g, Fiber: 10g, Sodium: 40mg

## *4. Sweet Potato Breakfast Hash*

**Ingredients:**

- One tiny sweet potato, chopped and peeled
- 1/4 cup diced bell peppers
- 1/4 cup diced onions
- 1 teaspoon olive oil
- Dash of garlic powder
- Dash of paprika
- Salt-free seasoning blend

**Preparation:**

1. Heat olive oil in a skillet over medium heat. Add diced sweet potatoes and cook until they begin to soften.
2. Add bell peppers and onions to the skillet. Sauté until vegetables are tender.
3. Season with garlic powder, paprika, and salt-free seasoning blend.

**Portion Size:** 1 serving

**Nutritional Information (approximate):**

Calories: 180 kcal, Protein: 3g, Carbohydrates: 30g, Fiber: 5g, Sodium: 60mg

## *5. Greek Yogurt Parfait*

**Ingredients:**

- 1/2 cup plain Greek yogurt (low-fat)
- 1/4 cup sliced strawberries
- 1 tablespoon chopped almonds
- 1 teaspoon honey (optional)

**Preparation:**

1. In a glass or bowl, layer Greek yogurt, sliced strawberries, and chopped almonds.
2. Drizzle with honey if desired.

**Portion Size:** 1 serving

**Nutritional Information (approximate):**

Calories: 180 kcal, Protein: 15g, Carbohydrates: 15g, Fiber: 3g, Sodium: 60mg

## *6. Whole Grain Toast with Avocado*

### Ingredients:

- 1 slice whole grain bread (low-sodium)
- 1/4 avocado, mashed
- 1 teaspoon lemon juice
- Pinch of black pepper
- Fresh herbs for garnish (optional)

### Preparation:

1. When the whole grain bread turns golden, toast it
2. In a bowl, mash the avocado with lemon juice and black pepper.
3. Top the toasted bread with a layer of mashed avocado.
4. Garnish with fresh herbs if desired.

**Portion Size:** 1 serving

**Nutritional Information (approximate):**

Calories: 150 kcal, Protein: 4g, Carbohydrates: 15g, Fiber: 5g, Sodium: 80mg

## *7. Berry Smoothie Bowl*

**Ingredients:**

- 1/2 cup frozen mixed berries
- 1/2 frozen banana
- 1/2 cup unsweetened almond milk
- 1 tablespoon chia seeds
- Toppings: sliced almonds, shredded coconut, fresh berries

**Preparation:**

1. In a blender, combine frozen berries, banana, almond milk, and chia seeds. Blend until smooth.
2. Pour the smoothie into a bowl and add toppings of sliced almonds, shredded coconut, and fresh berries.

**Portion Size:** 1 serving

**Nutritional Information (approximate):**

Calories: 250 kcal, Protein: 5g, Carbohydrates: 30g, Fiber: 10g, Sodium: 40mg

## Ingredients:

- 1/2 cup low-sodium cottage cheese
- 2 eggs
- 2 tablespoons oat flour
- 1/4 teaspoon baking powder
- Dash of cinnamon
- Fresh fruit for topping (optional)

## Preparation:

1. In a blender, combine cottage cheese, eggs, oat flour, baking powder, and cinnamon. Blend until smooth.
2. Heat a non-stick skillet over medium heat. Pour small amounts of batter onto the skillet to form pancakes.
3. Cook until bubbles form on the surface, then flip and cook until golden brown.
4. Serve pancakes with fresh fruit if desired.

**Portion Size:** 1 serving (3-4 small pancakes)

**Nutritional Information (approximate):**

Calories: 300 kcal, Protein: 25g, Carbohydrates: 15g, Fiber: 2g, Sodium: 180mg

*9. Veggie Breakfast Burrito*

**Ingredients:**

- 1 whole wheat tortilla (low-sodium)
- 2 eggs, scrambled
- 1/4 cup black beans (low-sodium, rinsed and drained)
- 2 tablespoons diced tomatoes
- 2 tablespoons diced bell peppers
- 1 tablespoon chopped cilantro
- Salsa or avocado (optional)

**Preparation:**

1. Warm the tortilla in a skillet or microwave.
2. Fill the tortilla with scrambled eggs, black beans, diced tomatoes, bell peppers, and chopped cilantro.
3. Roll the tortilla into
4. a burrito and serve with salsa or avocado if desired.

Portion Size: 1 serving

**Nutritional Information (approximate):**Calories: 300 kcal, Protein: 18g, Carbohydrates: 30g, Fiber: 8g, Sodium: 120mg

*10. Oatmeal with Berries and Almonds*

## Ingredients:

- 1/2 cup rolled oats
- 1 cup unsweetened almond milk
- 1/4 cup mixed berries (blueberries, strawberries)
- 1 tablespoon chopped almonds
- 1 teaspoon honey (optional)

## Preparation:

1. In a saucepan, combine rolled oats and almond milk. Bring to a boil, then reduce heat and simmer for 5-7 minutes until oats are cooked and mixture thickens.
2. Transfer the cooked oatmeal to a bowl and top with mixed berries and chopped almonds.
3. Drizzle with honey if desired.

**Portion Size:** 1 serving

**Nutritional Information (approximate):**

Calories: 250 kcal, Protein: 8g, Carbohydrates: 35g, Fiber: 7g, Sodium: 50mg

# Nourishing Low-Potassium Lunch Ideas:

*1. Grilled Chicken Salad*

**Ingredients:**

- 3 oz grilled chicken breast, sliced
- Mixed greens (lettuce, spinach)
- 1/4 cup sliced cucumbers
- 1/4 cup cherry tomatoes, halved
- 1 tablespoon balsamic vinaigrette (low-sodium)

**Preparation:**

1. Arrange mixed greens on a plate.
2. Top with grilled chicken slices, sliced cucumbers, and cherry tomatoes.
3. Drizzle with balsamic vinaigrette.

**Portion Size:** 1 serving

**Nutritional Information (approximate):**

Calories: 250 kcal, Protein: 30g, Carbohydrates: 8g, Fiber: 2g, Potassium: 250mg

## *2. Tuna Salad Wrap*

**Ingredients:**

- 3 oz canned tuna (in water, drained)
- 1 tablespoon plain Greek yogurt (low-fat)
- 1 tablespoon diced celery
- 1 tablespoon diced red onion
- Whole grain tortilla (low-sodium)
- Lettuce leaves

**Preparation:**

1. In a bowl, mix canned tuna, Greek yogurt, diced celery, and red onion.
2. Spread the tuna mixture onto a whole grain tortilla.
3. Top with lettuce leaves and roll into a wrap.

**Portion Size:** 1 serving

**Nutritional Information (approximate):**

Calories: 280 kcal, Protein: 25g, Carbohydrates: 20g, Fiber: 5g, Potassium: 280mg

*3. Veggie Stir-Fry with Brown Rice*

**Ingredients:**

- 1/2 cup cooked brown rice
- One cup of mixed veggies, such as carrots, bell peppers, and broccoli
- 2 tablespoons low-sodium stir-fry sauce
- 1 teaspoon sesame oil

**Preparation:**

1. Heat sesame oil in a pan. Add mixed vegetables and stir-fry until tender.
2. Add low-sodium stir-fry sauce and cook for an additional minute.
3. Serve stir-fried vegetables over cooked brown rice.

**Portion Size:** 1 serving

**Nutritional Information (approximate):**

Calories: 300 kcal, Protein: 8g, Carbohydrates: 50g, Fiber: 8g, Potassium: 300mg

*4. Turkey and Avocado Wrap*

## Ingredients:

- 3 oz roasted turkey breast, sliced
- 1/4 avocado, sliced
- Whole grain tortilla (low-sodium)
- Lettuce leaves
- Mustard or low-sodium dressing (optional)

## Preparation:

1. Lay out a whole grain tortilla.
2. Layer roasted turkey slices, avocado slices, and lettuce leaves.
3. Drizzle with mustard or low-sodium dressing if desired, then roll into a wrap.

**Portion Size:** 1 serving

**Nutritional Information (approximate):**

Calories: 280 kcal, Protein: 30g, Carbohydrates: 20g, Fiber: 5g, Potassium: 260mg

## 5. Egg Salad Lettuce Wraps

### Ingredients:

- 2 hard-boiled eggs, chopped
- 1 tablespoon plain Greek yogurt (low-fat)
- 1 teaspoon Dijon mustard
- Lettuce leaves
- Sliced radishes (optional)

### Preparation:

1. In a bowl, mix chopped hard-boiled eggs, Greek yogurt, and Dijon mustard.
2. Spoon the egg salad onto lettuce leaves.
3. Add sliced radishes for extra crunch if desired.

**Portion Size:** 1 serving

**Nutritional Information (approximate):**

Calories: 200 kcal, Protein: 14g, Carbohydrates: 4g, Fiber: 1g, Potassium: 200mg

## *6. Lentil Soup*

**Ingredients:**

- 1/2 cup dried lentils
- 2 cups low-sodium vegetable broth
- 1/4 cup diced carrots
- 1/4 cup diced celery
- 1/4 cup diced onions
- Herbs and spices (bay leaf, thyme, black pepper)

**Preparation:**

1. Rinse lentils and combine them with vegetable broth in a pot.
2. Add diced carrots, celery, onions, and herbs/spices.
3. Bring to a boil, then simmer for 25-30 minutes until lentils are tender.

**Portion Size:** 1 serving

**Nutritional Information (approximate):**

Calories: 220 kcal, Protein: 15g, Carbohydrates: 35g, Fiber: 15g, Potassium: 280mg

## 7. Baked Salmon with Quinoa

**Ingredients:**

- 3 oz baked salmon fillet
- 1/2 cup cooked quinoa
- 1/4 cup steamed green beans
- Lemon wedge for garnish

**Preparation:**

1. Bake salmon fillet seasoned with herbs or lemon juice until cooked.
2. Serve the baked salmon with cooked quinoa and steamed green beans.
3. Garnish with a lemon wedge for added flavor.

**Portion Size:** 1 serving

**Nutritional Information (approximate):**

Calories: 300 kcal, Protein: 25g, Carbohydrates: 20g, Fiber: 3g, Potassium: 300mg

## 8. Chickpea and Vegetable Salad

**Ingredients:**

- Half a cup of rinsed and drained canned chickpeas
- 1/4 cup diced bell peppers
- 1/4 cup diced cucumber
- 2 tablespoons chopped parsley
- 1 tablespoon lemon juice
- 1 teaspoon olive oil

**Preparation:**

1. In a bowl, combine chickpeas, bell peppers, cucumber, parsley, lemon juice, and olive oil.
2. Toss until well mixed and serve chilled.

**Portion Size:** 1 serving

**Nutritional Information (approximate):**

Calories: 250 kcal, Protein: 10g, Carbohydrates: 35g, Fiber: 10g, Potassium: 250mg

## *9. Shrimp Stir-Fry with Rice Noodles*

**Ingredients:**

- 3 oz cooked shrimp
- 1 cup cooked rice noodles
- 1 cup mixed stir-fry vegetables (bell peppers, broccoli, snap peas)
- 2 tablespoons low-sodium stir-fry sauce
- 1 teaspoon sesame oil

**Preparation:**

1. Heat sesame oil in a pan. Add stir-fry vegetables and shrimp, stir-fry until cooked.
2. Add cooked rice noodles and low-sodium stir-fry sauce. Mix well and heat through.
3. Serve hot.

**Portion Size:** 1 serving

**Nutritional Information (approximate):**

Calories: 320 kcal, Protein: 25g, Carbohydrates: 40g, Fiber: 5g, Potassium: 280mg

## *10. Chicken and Vegetable Skewers*

**Ingredients:**

- 3 oz grilled chicken skewers
- 1/2 cup grilled zucchini slices
- 1/2 cup grilled bell peppers
- 1/4 cup cooked brown rice (optional)

**Preparation:**

1. Thread grilled chicken, zucchini slices, and bell peppers onto skewers.
2. Grill until chicken is cooked through and vegetables are tender.
3. Serve with cooked brown rice if desired.

**Portion Size:** 1 serving

**Nutritional Information (approximate):**

Calories: 280 kcal, Protein: 30g, Carbohydrates: 20g, Fiber: 5g, Potassium: 300mg

# Flavorful Low-Phosphorus Dinners

## *1. Lemon Herb Baked Chicken*

**Ingredients:**

- 4 oz boneless, skinless chicken breast
- 1 tablespoon lemon juice
- 1 teaspoon olive oil
- 1/2 teaspoon dried herbs (thyme, rosemary)
- Salt and pepper to taste

**Preparation:**

1. Preheat oven to 375°F (190°C).
2. Mix lemon juice, olive oil, dried herbs, salt, and pepper in a bowl.
3. Marinate chicken breast in the mixture for 30 minutes.
4. Place the chicken in a baking dish and bake for 25-30 minutes until cooked through.

**Portion Size:** 1 serving

Nutritional Information (approximate):

Calories: 180 kcal, Protein: 25g, Carbohydrates: 1g, Fiber: 0g, Phosphorus: 150mg

## 2. Salmon with Dill Sauce

**Ingredients:**

- 4 oz salmon fillet
- 1 tablespoon plain Greek yogurt (low-fat)
- 1 tablespoon chopped fresh dill
- 1 teaspoon lemon juice
- Black pepper to taste

**Preparation:**

1. Preheat oven to 400°F (200°C).
2. Place salmon fillet on a baking sheet lined with parchment paper.
3. Mix Greek yogurt, chopped dill, lemon juice, and black pepper in a bowl.
4. Spread the dill sauce over the salmon and bake for 15-20 minutes until cooked.

**Portion Size:** 1 serving

**Nutritional Information (approximate):**

Calories: 250 kcal, Protein: 25g, Carbohydrates: 1g, Fiber: 0g, Phosphorus: 200mg

## *3. Turkey and Vegetable Stir-Fry*

**Ingredients:**

- 3 oz ground turkey
- 1 cup mixed stir-fry vegetables (broccoli, bell peppers, carrots)
- 1 teaspoon sesame oil
- Low-sodium stir-fry sauce

**Preparation:**

1. Heat sesame oil in a pan. Cook the ground turkey until it turns brown.
2. Add mixed vegetables and stir-fry until tender.
3. Drizzle with low-sodium stir-fry sauce and cook for an additional minute.

**Portion Size:** 1 serving

**Nutritional Information (approximate):**

Calories: 220 kcal, Protein: 25g, Carbohydrates: 10g, Fiber: 4g, Phosphorus: 180mg

## 4. Quinoa Stuffed Bell Peppers

**Ingredients:**

- Two bell peppers, cut in half and seeded
- 1/2 cup cooked quinoa
- 1/4 cup diced tomatoes
- 1/4 cup black beans (low-phosphorus)
- 1 tablespoon chopped cilantro
- 1/2 teaspoon cumin
- Salt and pepper to taste

**Preparation:**

1. Preheat oven to 375°F (190°C).
2. In a bowl, mix cooked quinoa, diced tomatoes, black beans, chopped cilantro, cumin, salt, and pepper.
3. Stuff the bell pepper halves with the quinoa mixture and bake for 25-30 minutes until peppers are tender.

**Portion Size:** 1 serving (2 stuffed pepper halves)

**Nutritional Information (approximate):**

Calories: 280 kcal, Protein: 10g, Carbohydrates: 50g, Fiber: 10g, Phosphorus: 150mg

**Ingredients:**

- 4 oz pork chops
- One tablespoon of finely chopped fresh herbs (thyme, rosemary)
- 1 teaspoon olive oil
- 1/4 cup breadcrumbs (low-phosphorus)
- Salt and pepper to taste

**Preparation:**

1. Preheat oven to 375°F (190°C).
2. Mix chopped herbs, olive oil, breadcrumbs, salt, and pepper in a bowl.
3. Coat pork chops with the breadcrumb mixture and place on a baking sheet.
4. Bake for 25-30 minutes until pork is cooked and crust is golden.

**Portion Size:** 1 serving

**Nutritional Information (approximate):**

Calories: 230 kcal, Protein: 25g, Carbohydrates: 10g, Fiber: 1g, Phosphorus: 200mg

## 6. Eggplant and Tomato Bake

### Ingredients:

- 1 small eggplant, sliced
- 1 cup diced tomatoes
- 1 tablespoon chopped basil
- 1 tablespoon grated Parmesan cheese
- 1 teaspoon olive oil

### Preparation:

1. Preheat oven to 375°F (190°C).
2. Arrange eggplant slices in a baking dish. Top with diced tomatoes and chopped basil.
3. Drizzle with olive oil and sprinkle grated Parmesan cheese.
4. Bake for 30-35 minutes until eggplant is tender.

**Portion Size:** 1 serving

**Nutritional Information (approximate):**

Calories: 150 kcal, Protein: 5g, Carbohydrates: 20g, Fiber: 8g, Phosphorus: 100mg

## 7. Chicken and Vegetable Kabobs

### Ingredients:

- 4 oz chicken breast, cubed
- 1/2 cup bell peppers, onions, and cherry tomatoes
- Low-sodium marinade
- Skewers

### Preparation:

1. Marinate chicken cubes in low-sodium marinade for 30 minutes.
2. Thread chicken, bell peppers, onions, and cherry tomatoes onto skewers.
3. Grill or bake until chicken is cooked and vegetables are tender.

**Portion Size:** 1 serving

**Nutritional Information (approximate):**

Calories: 200 kcal, Protein: 25g, Carbohydrates: 10g, Fiber: 2g, Phosphorus: 180mg

## *8. Lentil and Vegetable Curry*

**Ingredients:**

- 1/2 cup cooked lentils
- 1 cup mixed vegetables (cauliflower, carrots, peas)
- 1/4 cup diced onions
- 1 tablespoon curry paste
- 1/2 cup low-sodium vegetable broth

**Preparation:**

1. In a pan, sauté diced onions until translucent.
2. Add mixed vegetables and cook until tender.
3. Stir in cooked lentils, curry paste, and vegetable broth. Simmer for 10-15 minutes.

**Portion Size:** 1 serving

**Nutritional Information (approximate):**

Calories: 250 kcal, Protein: 15g, Carbohydrates: 40g, Fiber: 12g, Phosphorus: 180mg

## 9. Grilled Lemon Garlic Shrimp

**Ingredients:**

- 4 oz shrimp, peeled and deveined
- 1 tablespoon lemon juice
- 1 tablespoon minced garlic
- 1 teaspoon olive oil
- Black pepper to taste

**Preparation:**

1. In a bowl, marinate shrimp in lemon juice, minced garlic, olive oil, and black pepper for 15 minutes.
2. Grill shrimp until pink and cooked through.

**Portion Size:** 1 serving

**Nutritional Information (approximate):**

Calories: 150 kcal, Protein: 25g, Carbohydrates: 2g, Fiber: 0g, Phosphorus: 180mg

## *10. Mushroom and Spinach Pasta*

**Ingredients:**

- 1 cup cooked whole wheat pasta (low-phosphorus)
- 1/2 cup sliced mushrooms
- 1 cup fresh spinach leaves
- 1 tablespoon olive oil
- 1 tablespoon grated Parmesan cheese

**Preparation:**

1. In a pan, sauté sliced mushrooms until browned.
2. Add fresh spinach leaves and cook until wilted.
3. Toss cooked pasta with sautéed mushrooms, spinach, olive oil, and grated Parmesan cheese.

**Portion Size:** 1 serving

**Nutritional Information (approximate):**

Calories: 300 kcal, Protein: 10g, Carbohydrates: 40g, Fiber: 8g, Phosphorus: 150mg

# Kidney-Safe Snacks for Seniors

## 1. Apple and Almond Butter Slices

**Ingredients:**

- 1 medium apple, sliced
- 1 tablespoon almond butter (unsalted)

**Preparation:**

1. Slice the apple into wedges.
2. Spread almond butter on each apple slice.

**Portion Size:** 1 serving

**Nutritional Information (approximate):**

Calories: 150 kcal, Protein: 3g, Carbohydrates: 20g, Fiber: 5g, Sodium: 0mg

## *2. Rice Cake with Cottage Cheese*

**Ingredients:**

- 1 rice cake (low-sodium)
- 1/4 cup low-sodium cottage cheese

**Preparation:**

1. Spread cottage cheese on top of the rice cake.

**Portion Size:** 1 serving

**Nutritional Information (approximate):**

Calories: 100 kcal, Protein: 8g, Carbohydrates: 15g, Fiber: 1g, Sodium: 50mg

## *3. Carrot Sticks with Hummus*

**Ingredients:**

- 1 medium carrot, cut into sticks
- 2 tablespoons hummus (low-sodium)

**Preparation:**

- Serve carrot sticks with hummus for dipping.

**Portion Size:** 1 serving

**Nutritional Information (approximate):**

Calories: 80 kcal, Protein: 2g, Carbohydrates: 10g, Fiber: 3g, Sodium: 100mg

## 4. Greek Yogurt with Berries

**Ingredients:**

- 1/2 cup plain Greek yogurt (low-fat)
- 1/4 cup mixed berries (blueberries, raspberries)

**Preparation:**

- Serve Greek yogurt topped with mixed berries.

**Portion Size:** 1 serving

**Nutritional Information (approximate):**

Calories: 100 kcal, Protein: 12g, Carbohydrates: 10g, Fiber: 2g, Sodium: 50mg

## 5. Popcorn

**Ingredients:**

- 2 cups air-popped popcorn

**Preparation:**

- Air-pop popcorn and enjoy as a light snack.

**Portion Size:** 1 serving

**Nutritional Information (approximate):**

Calories: 60 kcal, Protein: 2g, Carbohydrates: 15g, Fiber: 3g, Sodium: 0mg

## 6. Celery Sticks with Peanut Butter

**Ingredients:**

- 2 celery stalks, cut into sticks
- 2 tablespoons peanut butter (unsalted)

**Preparation:**

- Spread peanut butter on celery sticks.

**Portion Size:** 1 serving

**Nutritional Information (approximate):**

Calories: 180 kcal, Protein: 6g, Carbohydrates: 8g, Fiber: 4g, Sodium: 0mg

## 7. Cottage Cheese and Pineapple Cubes

**Ingredients:**

- 1/2 cup low-sodium cottage cheese
- 1/4 cup pineapple cubes (fresh or canned in juice)

**Preparation:**

- Serve cottage cheese topped with pineapple cubes.

**Portion Size:** 1 serving

**Nutritional Information (approximate):**

Calories: 120 kcal, Protein: 14g, Carbohydrates: 15g, Fiber: 1g, Sodium: 100mg

*8. Kale Chips*

**Ingredients:**

- 2 cups kale leaves, torn into bite-sized pieces
- 1 tablespoon olive oil
- Salt-free seasoning blend

**Preparation:**

1. Preheat oven to 350°F (175°C).
2. Toss kale leaves with olive oil and salt-free seasoning.
3. Spread on a baking sheet and bake for 10-15 minutes until crispy.

**Portion Size:** 1 serving

**Nutritional Information (approximate):**

Calories: 50 kcal, Protein: 2g, Carbohydrates: 5g, Fiber: 2g, Sodium: 20mg

## *9. Sliced Cucumber with Tzatziki*

**Ingredients:**

- 1 medium cucumber, sliced
- 2 tablespoons tzatziki sauce (low-sodium)

**Preparation:**

- Serve cucumber slices with tzatziki for dipping.

**Portion Size:** 1 serving

**Nutritional Information (approximate):**

Calories: 40 kcal, Protein: 1g, Carbohydrates: 5g, Fiber: 1g, Sodium: 50mg

## Ingredients:

- 2 hard-boiled eggs

## Preparation:

- Boil eggs until cooked through and enjoy as a snack.

**Portion Size:** 1 serving

**Nutritional Information (approximate):**

Calories: 140 kcal, Protein: 12g, Carbohydrates: 1g, Fiber: 0g, Sodium: 120mg

# Low-Sodium and Low-Potassium Treats:

*1. Baked Apple Chips*

**Ingredients:**

- 2 apples, thinly sliced
- Cinnamon (optional)

**Preparation:**

1. Preheat oven to 200°F (95°C).
2. Place apple slices on a baking sheet lined with parchment paper.
3. Sprinkle with cinnamon if desired.
4. Bake for 1.5-2 hours until crispy, flipping slices halfway through.

**Portion Size:** 1 serving

**Nutritional Information (approximate):**

Calories: 50 kcal, Protein: 0g, Carbohydrates: 15g, Fiber: 3g, Sodium: 0mg, Potassium: 100mg

## *2. Frozen Banana Bites*

**Ingredients:**

- 2 bananas, sliced
- 1/4 cup dark chocolate chips (low-sodium)
- 1 tablespoon chopped nuts (optional)

**Preparation:**

1. Place banana slices on a parchment-lined tray.
2. Melt chocolate chips and drizzle over the bananas.
3. Optionally, sprinkle with chopped nuts.
4. Freeze until chocolate hardens.

**Portion Size:** 1 serving

**Nutritional Information (approximate):**

Calories: 90 kcal, Protein: 1g, Carbohydrates: 20g, Fiber: 2g, Sodium: 0mg, Potassium: 200mg

*3. Berry Sorbet*

## Ingredients:

- One cup of mixed berries, including raspberries, blueberries, and strawberries
- 2 tablespoons honey (optional)
- 1/4 cup water

## Preparation:

1. Blend berries, honey, and water until smooth.
2. Pour into a shallow dish and freeze for 2-3 hours, stirring occasionally for a slushy texture.

**Portion Size:** 1 serving

**Nutritional Information (approximate):**

Calories: 70 kcal, Protein: 1g, Carbohydrates: 18g, Fiber: 4g, Sodium: 0mg, Potassium: 100mg

## Ingredients:

- 1/2 cup plain Greek yogurt (low-sodium)
- 1/4 cup granola (low-sodium)
- 1/4 cup mixed berries

## Preparation:

- Layer yogurt, granola, and berries in a glass or bowl.

**Portion Size:** 1 serving

## Nutritional Information (approximate):

Calories: 150 kcal, Protein: 8g, Carbohydrates: 25g, Fiber: 3g, Sodium: 50mg, Potassium: 150mg

## *5. Rice Pudding*

**Ingredients:**

- 1/2 cup cooked white rice
- 1 cup unsweetened almond milk
- 1 tablespoon honey (optional)
- Cinnamon (optional)

**Preparation:**

1. In a saucepan, simmer rice, almond milk, and honey for 20-25 minutes until thickened.
2. Sprinkle with cinnamon if desired before serving.

**Portion Size:** 1 serving

**Nutritional Information (approximate):**

Calories: 120 kcal, Protein: 2g, Carbohydrates: 25g, Fiber: 1g, Sodium: 80mg, Potassium: 40mg

# 6. Mango Coconut Popsicles

## Ingredients:

- 1 ripe mango, peeled and diced
- 1/2 cup coconut water

## Preparation:

1. Blend mango and coconut water until smooth.
2. Pour into popsicle molds and freeze until solid.

**Portion Size:** 1 serving

**Nutritional Information (approximate):**

Calories: 80 kcal, Protein: 1g, Carbohydrates: 20g, Fiber: 2g, Sodium: 25mg, Potassium: 200mg

## 7. Chia Seed Pudding

**Ingredients:**

- 2 tablespoons chia seeds
- 1/2 cup unsweetened almond milk
- 1/2 teaspoon vanilla extract
- 1 teaspoon honey (optional)
- Sliced strawberries (optional)

**Preparation:**

1. In a bowl, combine chia seeds, almond milk, honey, and vanilla extract.
2. Refrigerate for at least 2 hours or overnight until it thickens.
3. Top with sliced strawberries if desired.

**Portion Size:** 1 serving

**Nutritional Information (approximate):**

Calories: 120 kcal, Protein: 4g, Carbohydrates: 10g, Fiber: 7g, Sodium: 50mg, Potassium: 90mg

## 8. Pineapple Coconut Ice Cream

**Ingredients:**

- 1 cup frozen pineapple chunks
- 1/2 cup coconut milk (unsweetened)
- 1 tablespoon shredded coconut (unsweetened)

**Preparation:**

1. Blend frozen pineapple and coconut milk until creamy.
2. Garnish with shredded coconut before serving.

**Portion Size:** 1 serving

**Nutritional Information (approximate):**

Calories: 120 kcal, Protein: 1g, Carbohydrates: 15g, Fiber: 2g, Sodium: 0mg, Potassium: 150mg

*9. Avocado Chocolate Mousse*

**Ingredients:**

- 1 ripe avocado
- 2 tablespoons cocoa powder (unsweetened)
- 2 tablespoons honey (optional)
- 1/4 cup unsweetened almond milk

**Preparation:**

1. Blend avocado, cocoa powder, honey, and almond milk until smooth.
2. Refrigerate before serving.

**Portion Size:** 1 serving

**Nutritional Information (approximate):**

Calories: 160 kcal, Protein: 2g, Carbohydrates: 15g, Fiber: 7g, Sodium: 10mg, Potassium: 450mg

## 10. Watermelon Slush

**Ingredients:**

- 2 cups diced watermelon (seedless)
- Juice of 1 lime
- Mint leaves (optional)

**Preparation:**

1. Blend watermelon and lime juice until smooth.
2. Pour into a shallow dish and freeze for 2-3 hours, stirring occasionally for a slushy texture.

**Portion Size:** 1 serving

**Nutritional Information (approximate):**

Calories: 60 kcal, Protein: 1g, Carbohydrates: 15g, Fiber: 1g, Sodium: 0mg, Potassium: 200mg

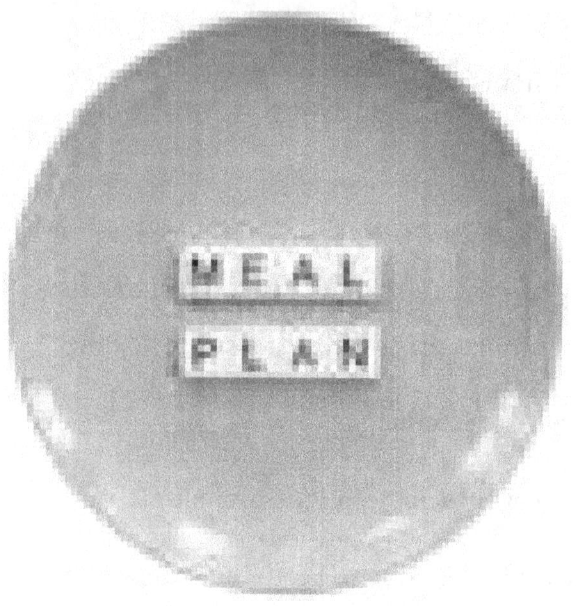
MEAL
PLAN

### DAY 1

BREAKFAST: Quinoa Breakfast Bowl

LUNCH: Chicken and Vegetable Skewers

DINNER: Lemon Herb Baked Chicken

SNACK: Hard-Boiled Eggs

DESSERT: Baked Apple Chips

### DAY 2

BREAKFAST: Veggie Omelette

LUNCH: Shrimp Stir-Fry with Rice Noodles

DINNER: Salmon with Dill Sauce

SNACK: Sliced Cucumber with Tzatziki

DESSERT: Frozen Banana Bites

### DAY 3

BREAKFAST: Overnight Chia Pudding

LUNCH: Chickpea and Vegetable Salad

DINNER: Turkey and Vegetable Stir-Fry

SNACK: Kale Chips

DESSERT: Berry Sorbet

## DAY 4

BREAKFAST: Sweet Potato Breakfast Hash

LUNCH: Baked Salmon with Quinoa

DINNER: Quinoa Stuffed Bell Peppers

SNACK: Cottage Cheese and Pineapple Cubes

DESSERT: Yogurt Parfait

## DAY 5

BREAKFAST: Greek Yogurt Parfait

LUNCH:  Lentil Soup

DINNER: Baked Herb-Crusted Pork Chops

SNACK: Celery Sticks with Peanut Butter

DESSERT: Rice Pudding

## DAY 6

BREAKFAST: Whole Grain Toast with Avocado

LUNCH: Egg Salad Lettuce Wraps

DINNER: Eggplant and Tomato Bake

SNACK: Popcorn

DESSERT: Mango Coconut Popsicles

## DAY 7

BREAKFAST: Berry Smoothie Bowl

LUNCH: Turkey and Avocado Wrap

DINNER: Chicken and Vegetable Kabobs

SNACK: Greek Yogurt with Berries

DESSERT: Chia Seed Pudding

## DAY 8

BREAKFAST: Cottage Cheese Pancakes

LUNCH: Veggie Stir-Fry with Brown Rice

DINNER: Lentil and Vegetable Curry

SNACK: Carrot Sticks with Hummus

DESSERT: Pineapple Coconut Ice Cream

## DAY 9

BREAKFAST: Veggie Breakfast Burrito

LUNCH: Tuna Salad Wrap

DINNER: Grilled Lemon Garlic Shrimp

SNACK: Rice Cake with Cottage Cheese

DESSERT: Avocado Chocolate Mousse

# DAY 10

BREAKFAST: Oatmeal with Berries and Almonds

LUNCH: Grilled Chicken Salad

DINNER: Mushroom and Spinach Pasta

SNACK: Apple and Almond Butter Slices

DESSERT: Watermelon Slush

# DAY 11

BREAKFAST: Quinoa Breakfast Bowl

LUNCH: Chicken and Vegetable Skewers

DINNER: Lemon Herb Baked Chicken

SNACK: Hard-Boiled Eggs

DESSERT: Baked Apple Chips

# DAY 12

BREAKFAST: Veggie Omelette

LUNCH: Shrimp Stir-Fry with Rice Noodles

DINNER: Salmon with Dill Sauce

SNACK: Sliced Cucumber with Tzatziki

DESSERT: Frozen Banana Bites

## DAY 13

BREAKFAST: Overnight Chia Pudding

LUNCH: Chickpea and Vegetable Salad

DINNER: Turkey and Vegetable Stir-Fry

SNACK: Kale Chips

DESSERT: Berry Sorbet

## DAY 14

BREAKFAST: Sweet Potato Breakfast Hash

LUNCH: Baked Salmon with Quinoa

DINNER: Quinoa Stuffed Bell Peppers

SNACK: Cottage Cheese and Pineapple Cubes

DESSERT: Yogurt Parfait

## DAY 15

BREAKFAST: Greek Yogurt Parfait

LUNCH:  Lentil Soup

DINNER: Baked Herb-Crusted Pork Chops

SNACK: Celery Sticks with Peanut Butter

DESSERT: Rice Pudding

## DAY 16

BREAKFAST: Whole Grain Toast with Avocado

LUNCH: Egg Salad Lettuce Wraps

DINNER: Eggplant and Tomato Bake

SNACK: Popcorn

DESSERT: Mango Coconut Popsicles

## DAY 17

BREAKFAST: Berry Smoothie Bowl

LUNCH: Turkey and Avocado Wrap

DINNER: Chicken and Vegetable Kabobs

SNACK: Greek Yogurt with Berries

DESSERT: Chia Seed Pudding

## DAY 18

BREAKFAST: Cottage Cheese Pancakes

LUNCH: Veggie Stir-Fry with Brown Rice

DINNER: Lentil and Vegetable Curry

SNACK: Carrot Sticks with Hummus

DESSERT: Pineapple Coconut Ice Cream

## DAY 19

BREAKFAST: Veggie Breakfast Burrito

LUNCH: Tuna Salad Wrap

DINNER: Grilled Lemon Garlic Shrimp

SNACK: Rice Cake with Cottage Cheese

DESSERT: Avocado Chocolate Mousse

## DAY 20

BREAKFAST: Oatmeal with Berries and Almonds

LUNCH: Grilled Chicken Salad

DINNER: Mushroom and Spinach Pasta

SNACK: Apple and Almond Butter Slices

DESSERT: Watermelon Slush

## DAY 21

BREAKFAST: Quinoa Breakfast Bowl

LUNCH: Chicken and Vegetable Skewers

DINNER: Lemon Herb Baked Chicken

SNACK: Hard-Boiled Eggs

DESSERT: Baked Apple Chips

# DAY 22

BREAKFAST: Veggie Omelette

LUNCH: Shrimp Stir-Fry with Rice Noodles

DINNER: Salmon with Dill Sauce

SNACK: Sliced Cucumber with Tzatziki

DESSERT: Frozen Banana Bites

# DAY 23

BREAKFAST: Overnight Chia Pudding

LUNCH: Chickpea and Vegetable Salad

DINNER: Turkey and Vegetable Stir-Fry

SNACK: Kale Chips

DESSERT: Berry Sorbet

# DAY 24

BREAKFAST: Sweet Potato Breakfast Hash

LUNCH: Baked Salmon with Quinoa

DINNER: Quinoa Stuffed Bell Peppers

SNACK: Cottage Cheese and Pineapple Cubes

DESSERT: Yogurt Parfait

## DAY 25

BREAKFAST: Greek Yogurt Parfait

LUNCH:  Lentil Soup

DINNER: Baked Herb-Crusted Pork Chops

SNACK: Celery Sticks with Peanut Butter

DESSERT: Rice Pudding

## DAY 26

BREAKFAST: Whole Grain Toast with Avocado

LUNCH: Egg Salad Lettuce Wraps

DINNER: Eggplant and Tomato Bake

SNACK: Popcorn

DESSERT: Mango Coconut Popsicles

## DAY 27

BREAKFAST: Berry Smoothie Bowl

LUNCH: Turkey and Avocado Wrap

DINNER: Chicken and Vegetable Kabobs

SNACK: Greek Yogurt with Berries

DESSERT: Chia Seed Pudding

## DAY 28

BREAKFAST: Cottage Cheese Pancakes

LUNCH: Veggie Stir-Fry with Brown Rice

DINNER: Lentil and Vegetable Curry

SNACK: Carrot Sticks with Hummus

DESSERT: Pineapple Coconut Ice Cream

## DAY 29

BREAKFAST: Veggie Breakfast Burrito

LUNCH: Tuna Salad Wrap

DINNER: Grilled Lemon Garlic Shrimp

SNACK: Rice Cake with Cottage Cheese

DESSERT: Avocado Chocolate Mousse

## DAY 30

BREAKFAST: Oatmeal with Berries and Almonds

LUNCH: Grilled Chicken Salad

DINNER: Mushroom and Spinach Pasta

SNACK: Apple and Almond Butter Slices

DESSERT: Watermelon Slush

# TIPS FOR SUSTAINING A HEALTHY DIET WITH KIDNEY DISEASE

Maintaining a healthy diet while managing kidney disease is crucial for managing symptoms, slowing its progression, and supporting overall health. Here are some essential tips for sustaining a healthy diet when dealing with kidney disease:

**1. Monitor Sodium Intake:** Limiting sodium helps manage fluid balance and blood pressure. Opt for fresh foods over processed ones, read labels for sodium content, and season meals with herbs and spices instead of salt.

**2. Control Phosphorus and Potassium:** High levels of phosphorus and potassium can be harmful to kidneys. Avoid high-potassium foods like bananas and oranges, and control phosphorus by reducing intake of dairy, beans, and nuts.

**3. Monitor Fluid Intake:** For those with fluid restrictions, managing fluid intake is crucial. Be mindful of not just beverages but also high-water content foods like soups, fruits, and vegetables.

**4. Optimize Protein Intake**: Depending on the stage of kidney disease, protein intake may need adjustment. Consulting a dietitian helps balance the right amount of protein to maintain muscle health without overburdening the kidneys.

**5. Choose Kidney-Friendly Foods:** Incorporate foods that support kidney health, such as cauliflower, cabbage, red bell peppers, onions, garlic, and berries. These are lower in potassium and phosphorus.

**6. Cook Smart:** Certain cooking techniques can reduce potassium and phosphorus. Boiling or leaching vegetables before cooking can reduce their potassium content.

**7. Manage Portions:** Controlling portion sizes helps manage nutrient intake and reduces strain on the kidneys. Utilize smaller plates to visually control portion sizes.

**8. Stay Hydrated:** While fluid intake might be restricted, maintaining adequate hydration is essential. Consult a healthcare provider for recommended fluid limits and suitable choices.

**9. Regular Monitoring:** Regular check-ups, including blood tests, are vital to monitor kidney function, potassium, phosphorus, and other vital levels. Adjustments to the diet can be made based on these results.

**10. Seek Professional Guidance:** Consulting a registered dietitian experienced in renal nutrition is invaluable. They can tailor a diet plan specific to individual needs, ensuring the right balance of nutrients while managing kidney disease.

**11. Mindful Eating:** Focus on mindful eating habits by savoring and enjoying meals. Chewing food thoroughly aids digestion and absorption, easing the workload on the kidneys.

**12. Be Adaptable:** As kidney function changes, dietary needs may vary. Being flexible and adapting the diet accordingly is key to sustaining kidney health.

Navigating a healthy diet with kidney disease requires attention to detail and personalized guidance. By focusing on nutrient balance, portion control, and choosing kidney-friendly options, individuals can effectively manage their condition and support overall well-being.

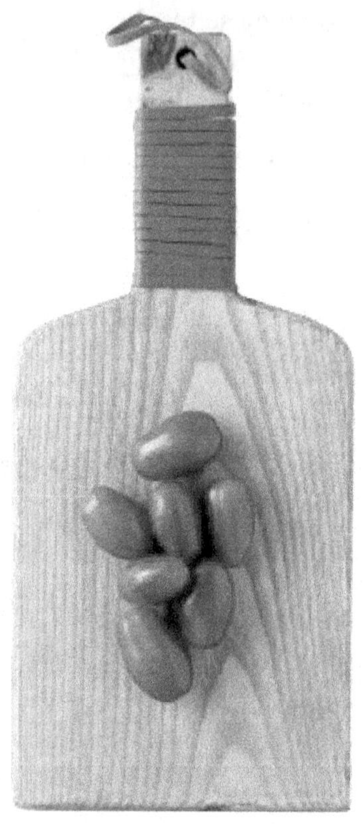

# CONCLUSION

Sustaining a healthy diet while managing kidney disease is a fundamental aspect of preserving kidney function and overall well-being. The journey to maintaining a kidney-friendly diet involves careful consideration of nutrient intake, portion sizes, and food choices.

By adhering to low-sodium, low-potassium, and controlled phosphorus diets, individuals can effectively manage symptoms, slow the progression of kidney disease, and maintain a better quality of life. Monitoring fluid intake, optimizing protein consumption, and incorporating kidney-friendly foods are vital strategies.

Professional guidance from a registered dietitian specializing in renal nutrition is invaluable. Their expertise in tailoring a diet plan specific to individual needs ensures the right balance of nutrients while adapting to changing kidney function.

Remember, it's not just about what one should avoid, but also about embracing mindful eating habits, staying hydrated within recommended limits, and being adaptable to evolving dietary requirements. Regular monitoring through check-ups and blood tests helps fine-tune dietary adjustments as needed.

Ultimately, a holistic approach to managing kidney disease involves a combination of medical care, lifestyle modifications, and dietary adjustments. By prioritizing a kidney-friendly diet, individuals can better manage their condition, support kidney health, and enhance their overall quality of life. Always seek personalized advice from healthcare professionals for the most effective and tailored dietary strategies suited to individual health needs.

# WEEKLY MEAL JOURNAL

WEEK ______________________    MONTH ______________________

### MONDAY

### SATURDAY

### TUESDAY

### SUNDAY

### WEDNESDAY

### SHOPPING LIST

### THURSDAY

### FRIDAY

### NOTES:

# WEEKLY
# MEAL JOURNAL

WEEK ________________    MONTH ________________

### MONDAY

### SATURDAY

### TUESDAY

### SUNDAY

### WEDNESDAY

### SHOPPING LIST

### THURSDAY

### FRIDAY

### NOTES:

# WEEKLY
# MEAL JOURNAL

WEEK _______________________     MONTH _______________________

### MONDAY

### SATURDAY

### TUESDAY

### SUNDAY

### WEDNESDAY

### SHOPPING LIST

- ○ _______________________
- ○ _______________________
- ○ _______________________
- ○ _______________________
- ○ _______________________
- ○ _______________________
- ○ _______________________
- ○ _______________________

### THURSDAY

### FRIDAY

**NOTES:**

- ○ _______________________
- ○ _______________________
- ○ _______________________
- ○ _______________________

# WEEKLY
# MEAL JOURNAL

WEEK _______________        MONTH _______________

MONDAY

SATURDAY

TUESDAY

SUNDAY

WEDNESDAY

SHOPPING LIST

THURSDAY

FRIDAY

NOTES:

# WEEKLY MEAL JOURNAL

WEEK _______________  MONTH _______________

MONDAY

SATURDAY

TUESDAY

SUNDAY

WEDNESDAY

SHOPPING LIST

THURSDAY

FRIDAY

NOTES:

# WEEKLY
# MEAL JOURNAL

WEEK ___________________    MONTH ___________________

### MONDAY

### SATURDAY

### TUESDAY

### SUNDAY

### WEDNESDAY

### SHOPPING LIST

### THURSDAY

### FRIDAY

### NOTES:

# WEEKLY MEAL JOURNAL

WEEK _______________________    MONTH _______________________

### MONDAY

### SATURDAY

### TUESDAY

### SUNDAY

### WEDNESDAY

### SHOPPING LIST

- ○ _______________________
- ○ _______________________
- ○ _______________________
- ○ _______________________
- ○ _______________________
- ○ _______________________
- ○ _______________________
- ○ _______________________

### THURSDAY

### FRIDAY

### NOTES:

- ○ _______________________
- ○ _______________________
- ○ _______________________
- ○ _______________________

# WEEKLY MEAL JOURNAL

WEEK ___________________  MONTH ___________________

| MONDAY | SATURDAY |
| TUESDAY | SUNDAY |
| WEDNESDAY | SHOPPING LIST |
| THURSDAY | |
| FRIDAY | NOTES: |